IMPROVE YOUR EYESIGHT

The best preventive guide to improving your eyesight with the use of simple exercises, vitamins, mineral, herbs, food and supplements for better vision; having no side's effect

BY

DOCTOR FRED BROWN

Copyright@2019

TABLE OF CONTENTS

CHAPTER ONE

EXPLAINING EYE MAINTENANCE

The eye is refers to as one of the most vital sense organ of the body which is usually for sight. With the assistance of eyes, reading, observing nature and the appreciation of art can be made possible. Enhancing the eyes with good cosmetics make it looks beautiful. Beautification of the eyes is carried out by wearing of simple sunglasses, hats; maintain better body weight, Avoid unwanted body stress and smoking.

Medicinal plant in their right proportion should be added to your daily eye maintenance plan. Any medicinal herbs (plants) you desire to take must be approved by Registered Health Organization in your state.

It is observed that some eye condition is not easily noticeable because it takes some time before the infection/disease could be seen. It is advise that you go for regular eye check/examination so as to detect eye diseases in their early stage and proffer solution to prevent loss of vision.

The brightness of the eyes is a topic of discuss in our society today since it is important for a healthy living. Several herbal food we eat contains the following; tinctures, teas and homeopathic eye drops. Speedy treatment to conjunctivitis is possible with the use of eye drops. The term conjunctivitis is refers to as irritation of the outer lining of the eyes thereby resulting to redness of the eyes and eye discharge.

It was discovered from research that this herbs removes diabetes (excessive sugar) from rat. It is the presence of diabetes in human that leads to eye problem.

SOME COMMON EYE DISEASES

a) CATARACTS

This is the presence of opacities in the lens of the eyes thus affecting your looking pattern through a water fall.

Factors that may cause cataracts are listed below;

- An older age
- Presence of Diabetes
- Smoking habit
- Excessive exposure to sunlight
- High intake of alcohol
- Nutrition Deficiency
- Excessive stress

- continuous usage of corticosteroids

b) GLAUCOMA

This is the inability to produce a draining fluid closer to the eyes thus causes pressure to build up, compression of optic nerve, tunnel vision and blindness.

c) MACULAR DEGENERATION

The retina is mainly affected in this case thereby creating difficulty in reading. Genetics factors may also be an issue. Below are some factors that can cause these diseases;

- Smoking habits
- High blood pressure
- Nutrition deficiency
- Excessive exposure to sunlight
- Excessive fat (Obesity)
- An older age

d) DIABETES RETINOPATHY

This is when the tiny blood vessels of the retina are destroyed by excessive blood glucose. A swollen of the blood vessels might be seen which will later leak off and later reform thereby causing difficulty in vision. High blood pressure causes diabetes retinopathy.

CHAPTER TWO

ACCEPTED HERBS FOR A HEALTHY EYE

1) GREEN TEA

It is called camellia sinensis and contains high level of antioxidants that gives free radicals. The high antioxidant present in the eyes will destroy any underlying diseases such like glaucoma, cataracts and macular degeneration.

Green teas polyphenols applications in the treatment of retinal cells protect the eyes from ultraviolet light that may cause cataracts and macular degeneration.

2) BILBERRY

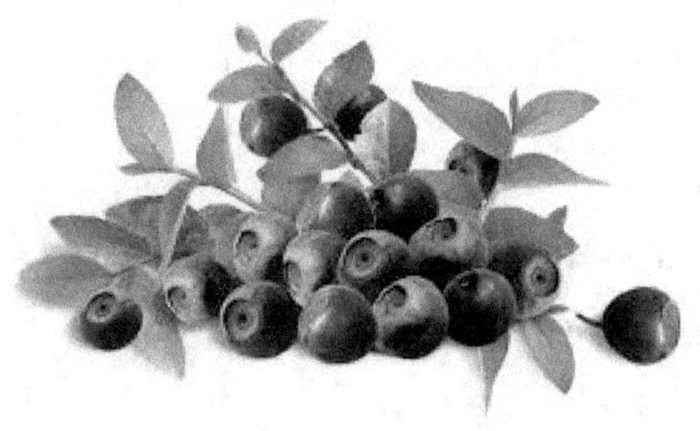

It is called vaccinium myrtillus. It contains potent antioxidant flavonoids which is sometimes called anthocyanins. It is botanical called Blueberry and cranberry in American. In the II world war, the Royal Air Force

Pilot said eating of bilberry herbs aid them with brighter vision.

A study since 1980s shows that bilberry herbs can manage the following challenges glaucoma, cataracts and diabetic retinopathy.

Studies are on going to show more importance of taking bilberry.

The list below shows some herbs, vegetables and fruits that have high level of antioxidant;

> Garlic
> Turmeric

- **GARLIC**

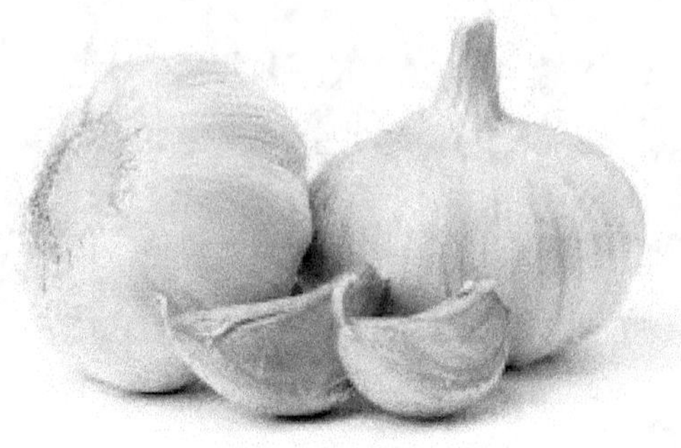

This is also called Allium Sativum. Findings gotten from several researches show that garlic can prevent cataracts.

- **TURMERIC**

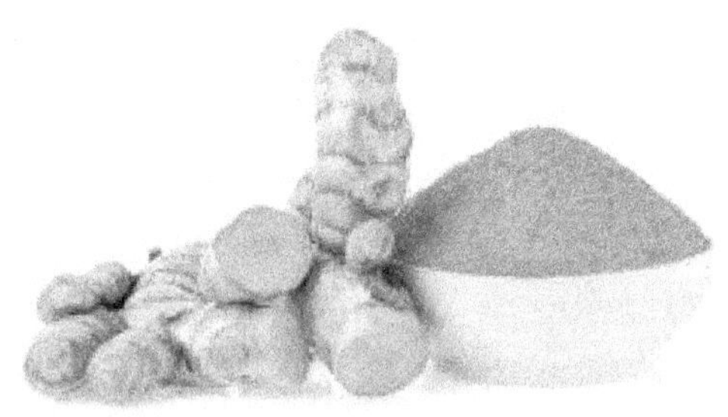

This is also called curcuma longa. Curcumin is the potent antioxidant residing in turmeric. Cataracts in rat can be destroyed with the application of Curcumin or with the addition of vitamin E.

See your medical practitioner immediately you notice an

unwanted symptom/pain in your eyes for onward advice.

3) GINKGO

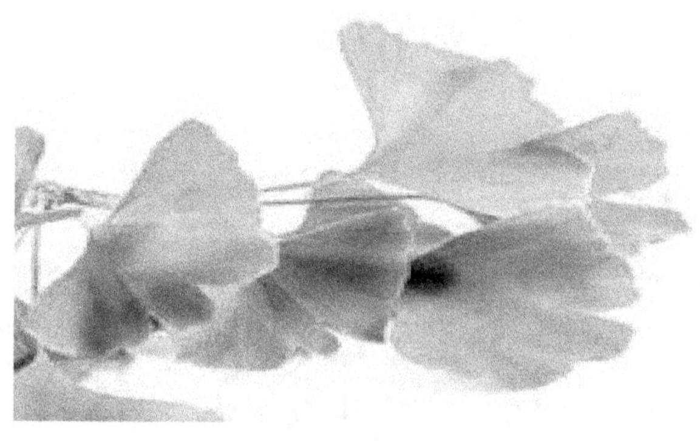

It is sometimes refers to as ginkgo biloba. It works well in the improving of blood flow to the retina. The retina is placed at the back part of the eye and it function is to sense the presence of light. The use of Ginkgo is to assist person suffering from glaucoma to get better vision. It is an antioxidant that protects the nerve cell and other vital cell connecting the eyes.

4) COLEUS

It is sometimes refers to as Coleus forskolin since it contains forskolin as part of it ingredient. Fluid formation within the eye will be reduced by the use of forskolin eye drops. This eye drop sometimes treatment glaucoma.

5) CANNABIS

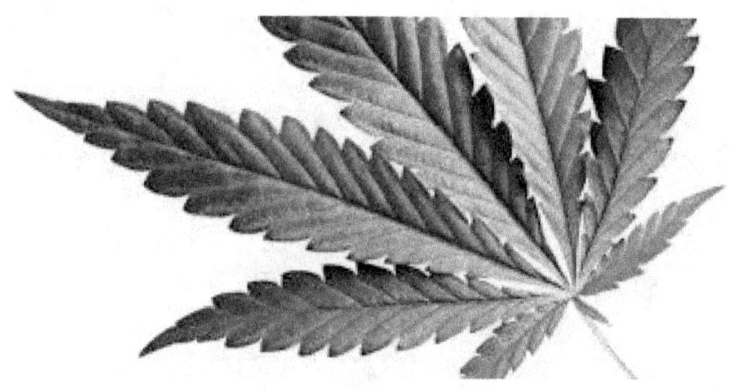

It is sometimes refers to as Cannabis savita. It contains cannabinoids as part of it ingredients which helps in reducing pressure found within the eyes. It works well for people having glaucoma. Cannabinoid can be taking by human through the following process;

I.   Inhaled
II. Intravenous
III. Oral intake

Side's effects to experience while taking cannabinoid are;

i.   Unbalanced mental state
ii. Presence of dry eyes
iii. Eyes color change to pink
iv. Blood pressure reduction

The treatment of eye diseases in some state/country are really challenging due to the fact that it is

not legally approved there to use
cannabinoid.

CHAPTER THREE

THE BEST VITAMINS FOR EYE HEALTH

Considering the vital role the eyes plays, vitamins and nutrients are needed for it to function well. These best nutrients and vitamins fight age-macular degeneration, cataracts, glaucoma and diabetic retinopathy.

Best vitamins for healthy eyes are listed below;

A.   VITAMIN A

Clear cornea is possibly achieved with the use of vitamin A. Cornea is known as an outer part that covers the eye.

Vitamin A has rhodopsin as its content which generates protein in the eyes so as to see clearly in low light environment.

Poor intake of vitamin A causes xerophthalmia. This disease condition begins in a gradual stage with night blindness. Continuous poor intake of vitamin A causes dry tear duct and dry eyes.

The dryness of tears and eye condition may cause softening of the cornea that might result to irreversible blindness. High intake of vitamin A will reduced the risk of getting cataracts and age-related macular degeneration.

Vitamins A diets are highly recommended for use than supplement for you to get clearer vision. Foods rich in vitamin A are sweet potatoes, leafy green vegetable, pumpkins and bell peppers.

B. NIACIN

Niacin can also be called vitamin B3. It helps in the breaking down of food eaten into useful energy. It is a good antioxidant.

Preventing glaucoma eye disease is best done with the application of niacin. Poor intake of niacin diets or supplements causes glaucoma.

Niacin supplement needs important direction for use before taking it so as to avoid the side's effects that may arise. 1.5 grams to 5 grams intake of niacin daily cause negative sides effect to the eyes. The effect includes vision looking blurred, inflammation of the cornea and damage of the macular.

Eating natural foods with niacin as the major content will not harm the eyes. Foods that contain niacin which are good for the eyes are listed below;

- ➢ Beef
- ➢ Mushroom
- ➢ legumes
- ➢ Poultry meat
- ➢ Fish
- ➢ peanuts

Note: the use of niacin helps in the prevention of glaucoma diseases. Take niacin supplement with caution to avoid been over

C. LUTEIN AND ZEAXANTHIN

Lutein and zeaxanthin are grouped as carotenoid family. Carotenoid is synthesized by plants.

Carotenoid exists in the retina and macula part of the eyes. It serves as filters that remove destructive blue light from damaging the eyes.

Carotenoid prevents cataracts. Lutein supplements Intake of 15 mg to 20 mg of will build up your vision if taken thrice daily for 5 months.

Since 6 mg of lutein and zeaxanthin yields better results, taking supplement may not be needed.

Lutein and zeaxanthin diets/food are vegetables and fruits. Collard greens, cooked spinach, and kale are very rich in carotenoids.

D.THE OMEGA -3 FATTY ACIDS

Omega -3 fatty acids is also termed polyunsaturated fat. It contains high level of DHA concentrated. The cells of the eye are protected with anti-inflammatory gotten from DHA thereby guiding against diabetic retinopathy.

Traditional Mediterranean diet known as oily fish might help prevent diabetic retinopathy.

If you have dry eyes challenges, omega-3 fat will help you generate more tears. The inability for the eyes to generate sufficient tears causes discomfort and partial blurry vision.

To get more omega-3 fatty acid in your body for better vision, daily meal must contain any of the following sources;

> Fish
> Flaxseed

➤ Chia seeds
➤ Nuts

E.   VITAMIN E

It is observed that most eye challenges are associated to oxidative stress. That is an imbalance condition that exists between free radicals and antioxidants resident in the body.

Vitamin E is an antioxidant whose aim is to protect the cells of the body and the eyes. These unstable molecules and free radicals resident in the body are there to fight vitamin E so as to gain access in attacking various cell of the body.

Here are some vital eye health nutrients highly rich in vitamin E; avocado, nut, seeds, leafy green vegetable, salmon and cooking oil. These diets will eliminate cataracts of the eyes. Vitamin E is also present in daily supplement called AREDS.

F. VITAMIN C

Vitamin C is a powerful antioxidant that suppresses any free radicals disturbing the eyes.

Vitamin C generates collagen (protein that gives the eyes especially the cornea and the sclera better structure). Cataracts are eliminated when vitamin C diets or supplements are in use. Fruits that contains vitamin C are listed below; "tropical fruits and citrus, broccoli, kale and bell peppers".

G.   VITAMIN B6, B9 AND B12

The combination of vitamin B6, B9 and B12 reduces the level of homocysteine in the body. Homocysteine is that protein resident in your body which is related to inflammation thereafter producing a risky AMD.

Important of vitamin B supplements is yet unknown.

H.RIBOFLAVIN

Riboflavin is sometimes called vitamin B2. It is a good antioxidant that aid speedy elimination of oxidative stress in the body.

Poor intake of vitamin B2 will tend to cause cataracts challenges.

An intake of 1.7 – 2.4 mg of riboflavin diets will help reduced the risk of getting cataracts.

Health professionals advise that 1.1 – 1.3 mg of riboflavin taken daily will help prevent cataracts. Fiboflavin diets are; beef, yogurt, oats, and fortified cereals.

I. THIAMINE

It is sometimes known for vitamin B1. It builds up body cell and converts food process into energy. It helps to fight cataracts occurrence. Thiamine diets helps to reduces cataracts by 40%.

Thiamine prevents early stage of diabetic retinopathy diseases in any person.

Clinical Research come up with a recommendation that taking thiamine for duration of three times daily; limit the existence of albumin present in your urine. Albumin present in your urine signifies diabetic retinopathy. These foods are rich in thiamine;

- Fish
- Meat
- Whole grains

You can add thiamine to your breakfast like;

- Cereals
- Bread
- Pasta

CHAPTER FOUR

BEST STEPS TO IMPROVE YOUR EYE SIGHT

1. ALWAYS STAY FIT

Regular exercise make your body fat burns out quickly thereby giving you healthy eyes. Overweight bring about Type 2 diabetes. This type 2 diabetes affects the tiny blood vessel that links the eyes. This condition is termed diabetic retinopathy.

High amount of sugar in your blood stream might injure the walls of the arteries. The small arteries in the retina are affected by excessive fat thereby allowing blood and fluid to gain access into the eye. Your vision will be negatively affected.

NOTE: make sure your blood sugar is regularly checked to remain fit always and prevent type 2 diabetes complications.

2. USE RULE 20-20-20

The eyes need rest after several uses during the day time. Working in front of a computer for very long time strains the eye. This strain can be ease by using rule 20-20-20.

"This rule implies you look at an object for 20 minute and such object is 20 feet away from you for every interval of 20 seconds.

3. DO AWAY WITH SMOKING

The Federal Ministry of Health warns that smoker is liable to die young. Smoking affects the following vital parts of the body;

- ➢ The Heart
- ➢ The Lungs
- ➢ The Skin
- ➢ The Teeth's
- ➢ The Eyes

Smokers are exposed to the following eye diseases;

- ➢ "Cataracts"
- ➢ "Age–related macular degeneration"

The moment smoking stops in your life, your damaging lungs, blood vessels, skin and eyes will start restoring to their original condition.

4. FID OUT ABOUT THE EYE HEALTH HISTORY OF YOUR FAMILY

Find out if the eye challenges you are having is hereditary from fathers or grandfathers. This step will guide you on how to solve the eye challenges

Below are some listed hereditary eye challenges;

> Optic Atrophy
> Age-Related Macular Degeneration
> Glaucoma
> Retinal Degeneration

With this useful information, preventing your eye challenges becomes easier.

5. YOU SHOULD CONTROL ANY CHRONIC CONDITION

Multiple sclerosis and high blood pressure are other health conditions that can also affect the eyes. It is termed chronic condition since it has the ability to affect your entire body.

The use of medication and balance diets that can help in managing multiple sclerosis since it can't be prevented.

High blood pressure can be prevented by the application of adequate exercise, balanced diets and medication that reduces hypertension.

6. USE A PROTECTIVE EYEWEAR FOR YOUR EYE

Get a good protective eyewear each time you are ready to go outside of your comfort place. Use your eyewear even when you are not doing risky work.

Your working environment determines the level of protection used for the eyes. Such risky environment can be chemicals, arc welding and a sharp moving object.

The eye protective goggles are design from polycarbonate which allows it to be tougher when compared to other plastics.

7. USE   PREFARED SUNGLASSES

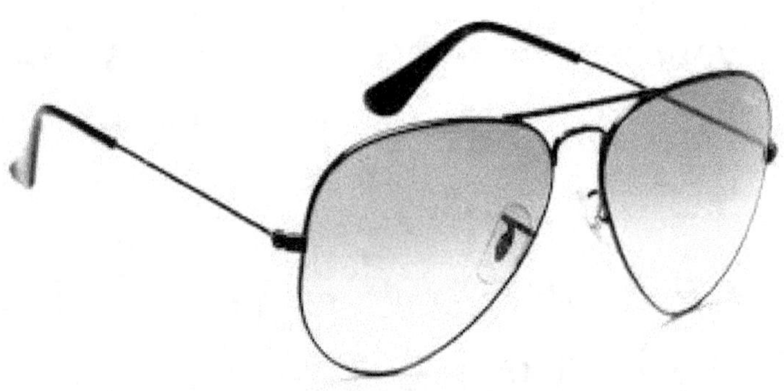

Sunglasses are not design only for dressing style purposes but also for the protection of the eyes.

Ultra-violet ray is prevented with the use of sunglasses.

The presence of cataracts and macular degeneration in the eyes can be prevented with the use of sunglasses.

The use of wide hat can protect the eyes from excessive shining of the sun.

8. GIVE YOUR HANDS AND LENSES BETTER HYGIENE

Human eyes are very delicate compare to other body parts. Germs and infections can easily affect the eye through the hand and lenses. Some things irritate the eye when it comes in contact with it.

Keep the hands neat by washing it with soapy water before coming in contact to the eyes and contact lenses. Disinfect your lenses as instructed by your medical personnel. Bacterial infection present in the eyes is caused by the presence of germs in the contact lenses.

CHAPTER FIVE

FOOD FOR A HEALTHY EYE

Recommended Nutrients for healthy eyes as stated by the American Optometric Association are seen below;

i.   CARROTS

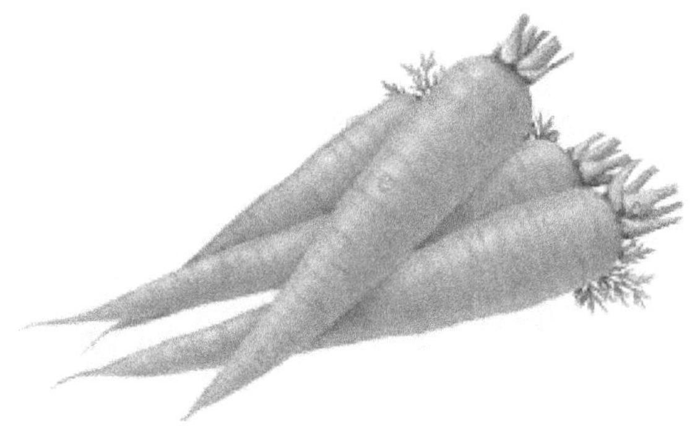

Carrots contain beta carotene and vitamin A. it is the presence of beta carotene present in carrots that makes the orange color to be visible.

Vitamin A is resident in protein which is refers to as rhodopsin. It helps to kill off light that is entering the retina.

ii. SWEET POTATOES

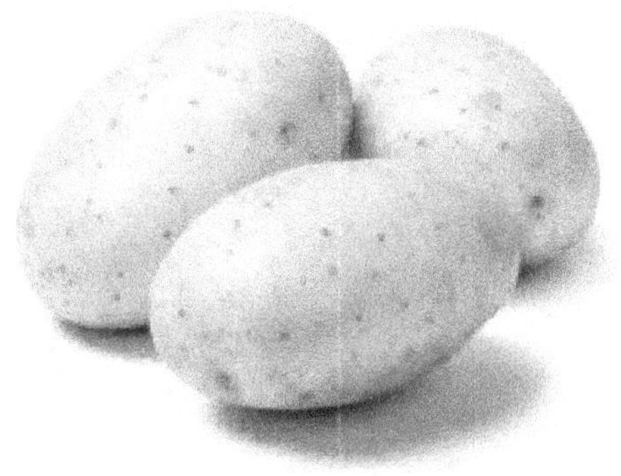

A sweet potato is an antioxidant vitamin E and rich in beta carotene.

iii.   BEEF

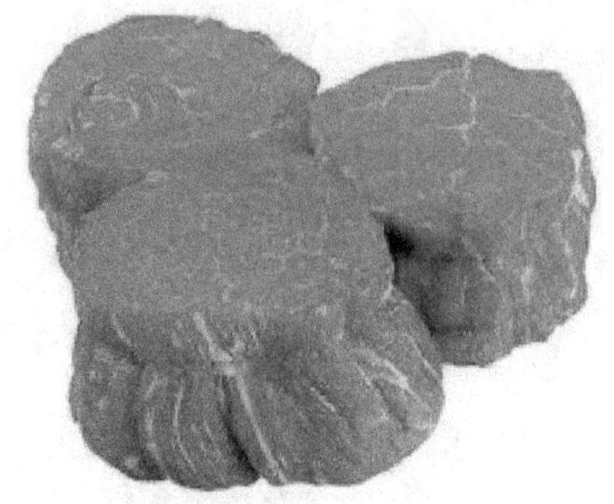

Beef is rich of zinc that aid delay in age-related sight loss or macular degeneration thereby giving a long lasting healthy eye.

The eye is normally high in zinc level such as the vascular tissue which is near the retina.

iv.   A FISH

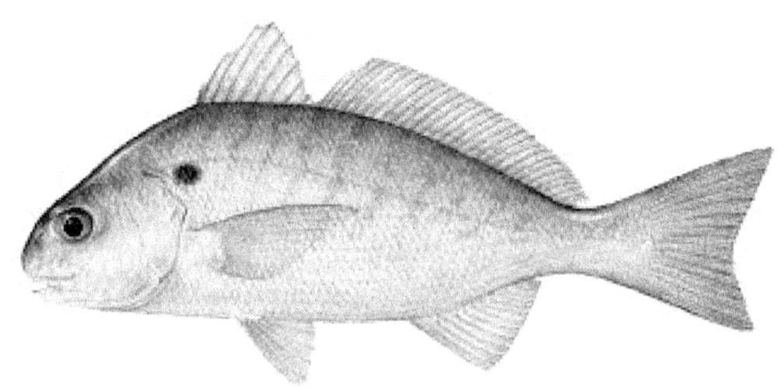

The following are needed to maintaining a healthy diets plan so as to keeps your eye from problems.

The Omega-3 fatty fish oil can be found in several fishes. The fishes reverse any condition of eye dryness. The fishes are listed below;

> Anchovies.
> The Salmon.
> The Tuna.
> Mackerel.
> Trout.
> The Herring.
> The Sardines.

v. NUTS AND LEGUMES

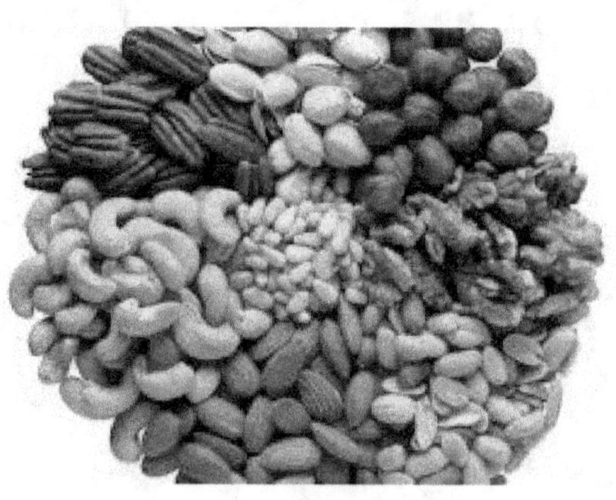

The Omega-3 fatty acid and the vitamin E are nutrient that is mainly gotten from nuts which protects the eyes against any form of age-related damages. Nuts are easily sold in any local super market close to your town. Below is the list of accepted nuts and legumes that will boost your vision;

- ➢ Peanuts.
- ➢ Walnuts.
- ➢ Cashews.
- ➢ Brazil Nuts.

vi.   SEEDS

Seed is another better source of vitamin E which is gotten easily from your local shops. Below are some of the seeds;

> The Hemp seeds.
> The Chia seeds.
> The Flax seeds.

vii.   THE CITRUS FRUIT

Citrus fruit is classified as a rich source of vitamin C. Citrus fruit are shown below;

> Orange.
> Lemons.

> Grape fruits.

viii.   THE GREEN VEGETABLE

The Green vegetable has in its content lutein and zeaxanthin. It is another good source of vitamin C. the green leafy vegetable can be gotten from the following;

> Collard.
> Spinach.
> Kale.

ix.   EGG

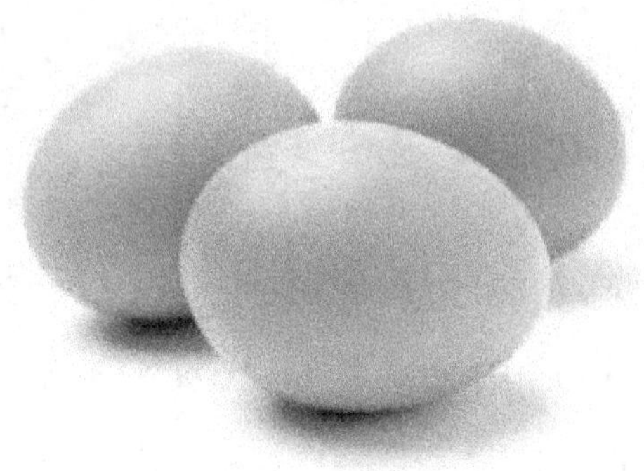

An egg is another source of lutein and zeaxanthin. Vitamin C, vitamin E and zinc is classified as important nutrient gotten residing in eggs. Age-related sight loss will be a forgotten issue with the right intake of egg.

x. WATER

Taking reasonable amount of water is good in building of the body. Dehydration is averted which thereafter reduces dryness of the eyes.

NOTE: For healthy eyes to be a reality here are the required nutrient that must be taken as recommended.

- ➢ Vitamin C = 500 mg.
- ➢ Vitamin E = 400 international units.
- ➢ Zinc oxide =80 mg.
- ➢ Copper oxide = 2 mg.
- ➢ Lutein =10 mg.
- ➢ Zeaxanthin = 2 mg.

CHAPTER SIX

EXERCISE NEEDED TO IMPROVE YOUR EYESIGHT

The eyes are made of muscles which when over used in one position can cause sore in the eye. Give a little rest to the eye muscle after prolonged use of the eyes.

Headache and glaucoma will be eliminated when the eye muscles are engaged in exercises. Special time is not needed to be devoted for this exercise. Here are the exercises needed to improve your eyesight;

1) PALMING

Rub your palms together toughly rub so as to generate heat. You will now place the warm hands on your eyelids so that the generated heat can be transferred to the eyes. Do these continuously for about 2 to 3 times till the eyes muscle become relaxed.

2) BLINKING

Get a good sitting position with your eyes clearly opened. Blink your eye for about 10 to 15 times. Relax with the eyes closed for about 20 seconds. Do this process for 3 to 4 times.

3) ZOOMING

This simply means making an object to come closer to your eye so that there will be a change in vision. Sit comfortably with the arms stretched forward and the thumb facing up. Carefully bend your arm so as to face the direction of your eye thereby making zooming of the thumb to be easy.

4) SHIFTING

This is slightly rotation of the eyeball from one location to the other. This process allows functioning spurt of blood to go to the eye muscle.

SUMMARY

Diabetes is known to be one main causes of blindness. Take your medications as prescribed by your medical doctor with adequate blood sugar level check.

Focus on better intake of low-moderate glycemic index with better control to carbon hydrate intakes.

Check on your optometrist or ophthalmologist to see if any eyesight challenges still exist so that quick treatment will be applied to the ailment.

THE END